Kathleen O'Bannon

Whole Foods
for
Seniors

Feel Younger!
Live Longer!

books

Vancouver
Canada

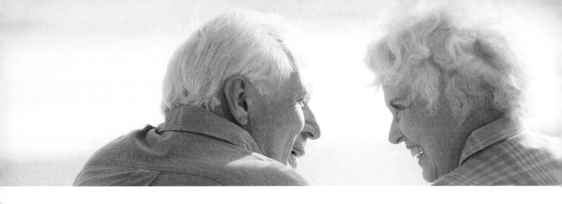

contents

Note: Conversions in this book (from imperial to metric) are not exact. They have been rounded to the nearest measurement for convenience. Exact measurements are given in imperial. The recipes in this book are by no means to be taken as therapeutic. They simply promote the philosophy of both the author and *alive* books in relation to whole foods, health and nutrition, while incorporating the practical advice given by the author in the first section of the book.

Recipes

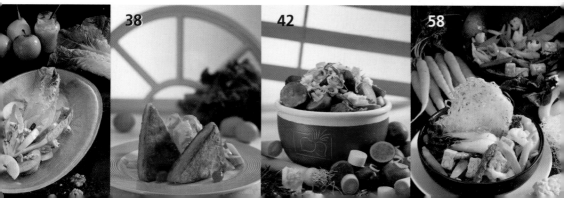

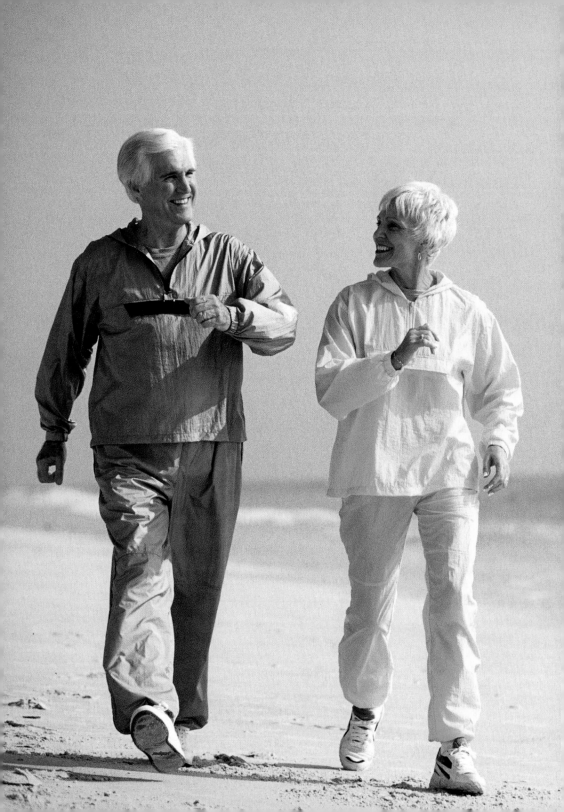

Whole foods can help restore vitality and energy in anyone at any age!

Whole foods contain the nutrients necessary to sustain life and give you energy. Processed foods do not.

Introduction

The dream of the 1940s, 50s and 60s was to retire and have enough health, wealth and time left to travel and enjoy life. For some people this has become a reality, but many seniors today suffer from health problems that prevent them from enjoying the "golden years" of retirement and aging. But it doesn't have to be that way.

You can start changing your health and your life today! Much of today's so-called foods offer empty calories and a load of additives. The taste, convenience and long shelf life are not a fair trade for your health. The more a food is altered, processed or packaged, the less nourishment it contains. Processed food and fast food is full of harmful trans-fatty acids, sugar and salt, and is lacking in fiber and enzymes. Meats contain residues of hormones and traces of medications that are fed to animals. Much of our produce has been sprayed with pesticides. It's no wonder, as our bodies age, that most of us feel tired and find ourselves fighting various ailments.

You can start feeling better today!

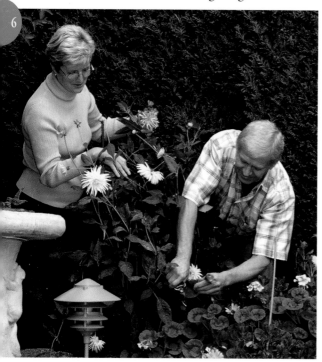

The fact is that successive years of eating highly-refined, over processed, pesticide-ridden foods can take their toll on even the strongest human. Even our most common diseases do not happen over night. They develop over the course of many years; they are degenerative diseases. Many diseases start quite simply. Over-consumption of refined oils and hydrogenated (artificially hardened) fats in combination with refined sugar and a lack of exercise lead to obesity, which is linked to cancer, diabetes, heart disease, high blood pressure and arthritis. It's true—strokes and arteriosclerosis are also the

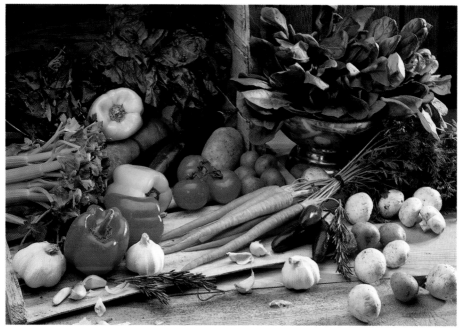

result of a poor diet. We are overfed, and undernourished. So why not ensure your diet is rich, not poor? Why not decide right now to put a stop to this self-destruction? It's not too late! Decide to eat whole foods—the foods your body wants and can thrive on.

The food choices you make will change your life and your health for the better.

A nutritious, whole-food diet is an integral part of preventing disease and maintaining health. Whole food is real food. And food in its natural, unrefined state contains valuable healing qualities. Nature provides the correct balance of nutrients for us. Hippocrates, the Father of Medicine, set a medical precedent in considering the role of nutrients in relation to health and disease. Centuries later, the modern medical establishment is starting to acknowledge the role dietary habits and nutrition play in creating disease.

Avoid So-Called "Aging Problems"

What are the benefits of a whole-foods diet? The end of heart-burn, acid reflux, postnasal drip, migraines, constipation, irritable bowel syndrome, prostate problems, menopause symptoms, low blood sugar, muscle stiffness and many other health problems that the media says you have to live with just because you are older. These and other problems will disappear when you begin to follow a whole-foods eating plan. The power of nutrients to prevent and cure disease is being researched around the world. There are substances in our food, long overlooked as not being important, that are now being discovered to have a healing effect. The phytonutrient lutein, for example, is found in kale and is shown to prevent age-related macular degeneration, which can cause permanent blindness.

Diabetes

There is an epidemic of blood sugar problems in North America brought on by refined food diets. A diet high in refined sugar or white flour can produce insulin resistance or insulin sensitivity, which is being treated with drugs. There is no need for this epidemic. The epidemic occurs from the huge number of people, children and seniors alike, who are eating nutritionless food and throwing off the precious balance of blood sugar and insulin in their bodies, leading to health problems such as diabetes. It is a logical cause-and-effect situation.

High glycemic foods, such as those that contain white sugar, throw off the balance of the body.

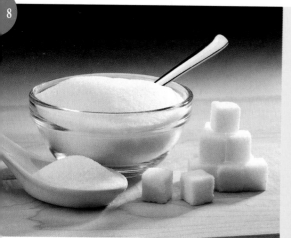

High Glycemic Foods

Our forefathers, eating a natural, whole foods diet, didn't need to concern themselves with details about glycemic indexes and so on. Their food contained all the elements that ensure proper digestion and absorption. All this has changed since the average diet now includes foods that are refined and fractionated–all for the increase of shelf life and financial profits.

The glycemic rating of foods tells you how fast the natural or refined sugars will enter your blood stream. The highest rating goes to white refined sugar. High glycemic foods tend to throw off the delicate balance in the body and cause rapid rises in blood sugar followed by rapid drops in blood sugars, often called hypoglycemia. This is not only hard on your body, but also dangerous. Staying away from refined sugars and flours can help you overcome this health problem before you join the statistics as a Type II diabetic. The National Institute of Diabetes and Digestive and Kidney Diseases (NIDDKD) says there are at least 16 million people in the United States who have diabetes, and about one third of them don't even know they have it.

Low Glycemic Foods

Low glycemic foods enter the blood stream slowly and have also been called "slow release" foods. Whole grains like brown rice, whole wheat, whole barley, millet, and quinoa are slow release and will not cause a sudden rise in blood sugar. Refined grains (white rice, pearl barley, white flour, and the products made from white flour like pasta, white bread, and cous cous) are quick release and can cause blood sugar fluctuations. When you eat a whole foods diet you will experience constant energy all day long, not the sudden raising and falling of energy and moods that come from eating refined foods.

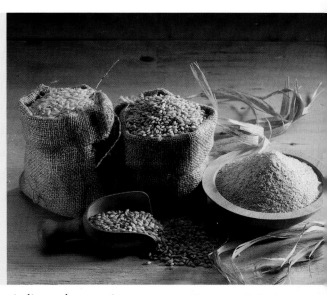

Whole foods can help restore vitality and energy in anyone at any age–even if you have been eating the typical North American diet of mostly refined white flour and sugar (white bread, white pasta, cookies, chips, boxed cereal and crackers, etc.); and refined oils (margarine, shortening and packaged foods). By changing to a whole-foods diet it is possible to feel better, be more alert, have fewer aches and pains, and even begin to reverse some of those nagging health problems you thought were a normal result of aging. Whole foods contain the nutrients necessary to sustain life and give you energy. Processed foods do not!

Low glycemic foods do not cause a sudden rise in blood sugar as high glycemic foods do.

You Really *Are* What You Eat

I have always said that you are like your food. If you want to be old, washed out, dull and dreary, eat processed, over-cooked, dull, dreary food. But if you want to be alive, vital and brimming with energy, eat vital, alive, whole foods. It's that simple. In the whole-foods revolution, we believe that many problems of aging and disease are due to faulty eating habits, poor food choices, sluggish digestion, and lack of exercise. You need to get back to the basics, which means re-training your taste buds. A healthy body desires whole foods. An unhealthy diet leads to cravings for refined flour products, sugar and junk food. Once you begin eating a whole-

The China Project

Dr. T. Colin Campbell, of Cornell University in Ithaca, New York, told me in an interview in 1990 that his China study (Diet, Lifestyle and Mortality in China: A study of the Characteristics of 65 Chinese Counties) showed that as people became more "civilized" and lived near or in large cities, their health became increasingly poor. This study showed that as they ate more refined white rice and less whole foods (brown rice) they suffered from the diseases of "civilized" people. People who lived in the more rural areas of China had none of the diseases of the wealthy. These diseases are various cancers, diabetes, heart disease and osteoporosis.

Osteoporosis was unheard of in the rural areas where they ate no dairy products and only consumed vegetable proteins or no more than 7% of their daily protein from animal proteins. All of their calcium came from vegetable sources like dark green leafy vegetables, sea vegetables and tofu. Cabbage is very rich in calcium and is easily absorbed. He estimated that the average rural Chinese woman ate about 400 mg of calcium in the form of food stuffs. And still they had no osteoporosis! The study reports that their conclusion for this is that they ate very little animal protein and animal fats. They ate whole foods! Health foods!

foods diet your taste for real food will return and processed and sugary foods will not be a natural choice for you.

I am a great example of what whole foods can do. I am a senior and have been eating whole foods since the 1960s. I feel great, have lots of energy and rarely get sick. This is not how I spent most of my youth and university years, however. I was always sick. I had bronchitis, tonsillitis, colds and every flu that came by, and felt half dead most of the time. I was twenty-five before I found out that healthy people don't blow their noses every day before getting out of bed. Everybody in my family did it; I had always done it. But when I changed to a whole-foods diet, I never had postnasal drip again.

When I was a child, we always had white bread; even the bread my mother made was white. We also had what I call "white death"–white sugar, and I drank a lot of artificially sweetened drinks then, too. My mother cooked what used to be called "English style:" everything was boiled to death. All the enzymes required for good metabolism were gone because they don't withstand heat of 118°F (48°C) or more. My heart goes out to today's young people who have grown up with processed foods and nothing else. Often, their medical records tell the story of what it's done to them. I know of a study conducted at a school where teenaged students were asked to record what they ate for sixteen days. Believe it or not a whopping 17 percent of them did not eat one piece of raw food (fruit or vegetable) the entire time. Everything they ate was cooked, and therefore depleted, or completely devoid, of enzymes.

Symptoms of Nutritional Deficiencies	
Symptom	**Nutrient Required**
Anemia	Iron, vitamin B_{12}, folate
Bleeding gums	Vitamin C, folate
Cardiac arrhythmia	Potassium, magnesium
Clotting abnormalities	Vitamin K
Dental decay	Fluoride
Dry, rough skin	Vitamin A
Goiter	Iodine
Growth problems	Zinc
Healing abnormalities	Vitamin C, zinc
Light sensitivity	Riboflavin
Liver damage	Vitamin K
Mental confusion, mood disorders	B vitamins
Mouth sores, inflammation	Riboflavin, niacin, vitamin B_6
Muscle cramps, wasting	Thiamine
Muscle weakness	Magnesium, potassium
Nerve damage	Vitamin B_{12}
Night blindness	Vitamin A
Psychosis	Thiamine
Reduced immunity	Vitamins A and C, zinc
Rickets; bone deformities	Vitamin D, calcium

Whole Wheat–Ugh?

One day in 1969 I had some friends over for dinner. The woman arrived early and helped me make–and eat–some doughnuts. She ate three and then asked me what they were made of. When I said whole-wheat flour and yogurt, she actually spat out what she was eating and said, "Whole-wheat flour–ugh!" Of course she had already enjoyed three of them! This was my first experience with people's food prejudices. She just "knew" she wouldn't like whole-wheat flour doughnuts and didn't want to eat them. I couldn't believe that she could be so stubborn. I would have expected her to say, "Wow! Whole-wheat flour! I would never have guessed."

Don't be like my friend. Have an open mind about whole foods. You might find that they are different, but you will like them. Your body was made to eat whole foods, but you have

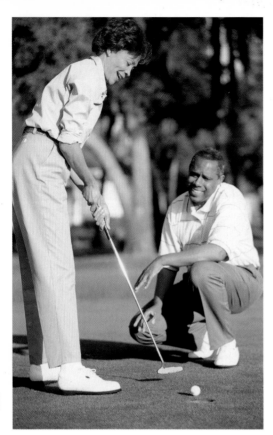

learned to enjoy food that is not good for your body. Imagine how much better food that is good for you will taste.

It's Never Too Late To Change

It's never too late to change your lifestyle for the better. I have seen people of all ages make the change to whole foods and feel younger and more vital as a result. I'm so glad you are reading this book and have decided to learn about whole foods. I have seen people reverse even diabetes in a few short months on a whole-foods diet. Heart disease, high blood pressure, heartburn, headaches, sore muscles and many other health problems can be reversed or improved by changing to a whole-foods diet. You can even start to look and feel younger. It's never too late to feel better, be more alert and have a glow of health about you.

Many health problems can be prevented, improved and reversed by switching to whole foods.

A Picture Is Worth a Thousand Words

When I worked in Toronto at the Nutritional and Preventive Medical Clinic, I had a client who, though she was only forty, came in suffering from headaches, backaches, low energy, lack of vitality and insomnia; she looked exhausted. I took a photograph of her. After about a month on a whole-foods program she returned for a check-up. I asked, "How are the headaches?" She replied, "What headaches? I don't have headaches." "How are your backaches?" "What backaches? I don't have backaches." She looked at me and said, "Are you sure you have my chart? I don't have those problems." I showed her the photograph of her when she first came to the clinic and she said, "That's not me, look how bad that woman looks." She had gotten rid of all her health complaints in a few weeks and had forgotten that she ever felt or looked that bad. Then she said, "You know, I feel so good, I'm thinking of trading my forty-year-old husband in on two twenty-year-olds!"

You can experience this kind of improvement too, by following a healthful lifestyle, including a whole-foods diet.

What are Whole Foods, Anyway? . . . .

Food is your body's fuel. If you put better fuel in your body it will run better. Think of how it would be if you ran a high-performance racecar on low-grade fuel. You wouldn't win many races. The same is true for your body. You can't expect your body to be in tip-top shape if you put in food that has little nutritional value–low-grade fuel.

Whole foods are alive and vital: they are top-quality foods, excellent high-grade fuel for your body. Whole foods are the fuel that your body was made to run on and it will run at peak performance all day long when you eat them regularly.

> ### Defining Whole Foods
> - The food must be the whole, unprocessed food–nothing has been taken away; it can be a food directly derived from a whole food, as long as the derivative contains all or most of the nutrients of the original.
> - The food contains no artificial substances–nothing has been added.
> - The food's effect on the health of the body is positive.

The Whole Food, and Nothing But the Whole Food

A whole food is, as the name implies, the entire food. This means it has not been processed, preserved, refined, frozen, canned, polished, bleached, peeled or otherwise stripped of nutrients. Why is it important to eat the whole food? Because there are more than fifty essential nutritional substances that you must consume for

good health. These include eight amino acids (proteins), carbohydrates, fiber, fats, two essential fatty acids, twenty vitamins, twenty minerals, and of course, water. If you don't eat whole foods, it is easy to miss some of these. Vitamin, mineral and other supplements are fine, but whole foods are better because they contain the perfect balance of everything you need to be healthy.

You wouldn't put bad fuel in your car, so why put harmful food in your body?

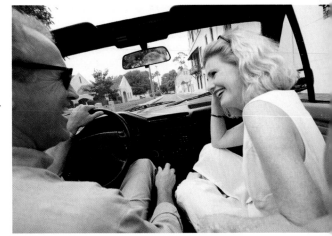

Let's look at an example of a whole food and why we need it. "Brown" rice is a whole food. White rice is not a whole food. Rice has many layers: the outer bran layer, which is high in fiber; the next layer, which has B vitamins in it; and then the starch inside. When the bran and B vitamins are removed (they are the brown part), you have white rice, which is just starch. Don't get me wrong; there is nothing bad about starch. However, your body needs B vitamins to fully digest the starch in rice. That's why they're naturally there in the first place! If you need B vitamins and they have been removed by polishing the rice, you have to get them from the rest of your meal. This means that each time you eat white rice, you need more than the usual amount of B vitamins from the rest of your meal to digest the starch in the rice. You could become deficient in B vitamins.

It's the same with wheat. Whole wheat contains all the B vitamins, enzymes and fiber needed to digest it. These are removed to make white flour. White flour is difficult to digest, robs your body of B vitamins and causes stress in your body. When there is stress in your body your digestion stops automatically. Does this sound like a vicious circle? It is!

When grains are refined, polished and denatured the bran is removed. The bran is there to provide fiber and improve the digestion of the food. Without the B vitamins and the bran, it is very difficult to digest rice, wheat and many other foods.

Beyond Rice and Wheat

Rice and wheat are not the only foods being denatured and passed off as "real" food. Barley and sugar are two others that are being processed. Whole barley is a whole food; pearl barley is processed and polished. Sucanat® and Rapadura® are two brands of whole sugar. They are sugarcane juice that has been dried and left whole. White sugar has had the B vitamins removed, resulting in a need for more B vitamins to break it down and digest it.

The most important minerals contained in raw cane juice or sugar beet juice are calcium and potassium. These are removed in the refining process along with iron (which gives the juice the brown color), magnesium and phosphorus. White refined sugar cannot be digested or metabolized if these minerals, especially the calcium, are not present. That is why the consumption of sugar first attacks the teeth where calcium is exposed and also the bones, causing a calcium-phosphorous deficiency leading to osteoporosis. It's as simple as that. Nutrient deficiencies are responsible for all degenerative diseases.

Eating whole foods means eating as much of the food in its natural state as possible. A baked potato with the skin on is a whole food; french-fried, peeled potatoes are not. Unpeeled, steamed potatoes are whole foods; peeled, boiled potatoes are not. Dark-green lettuce is a whole food; pale or white lettuce is not. Whole-grain pasta is a whole food; white-flour pasta is not. White bread is not a whole food, nor is 60 percent whole wheat bread. Only 100 percent whole wheat bread is a whole food, or other breads that are made with whole food ingredients. Apple pie with a whole-wheat crust, unpeeled apples and evaporated sugarcane juice or honey is a whole food; apple pie with a white-flour crust, peeled apples and white sugar is not—you get the picture!

There's a recipe for whole-food apple pie in the recipe section that will convince you to eat whole foods if nothing else does! Walnuts, hazelnuts, almonds and all kinds of different nuts, such as pumpkin, sunflower and flax are whole foods, as are the oils that come from them (if they're cold-pressed and unrefined, that is). The oils, when refined, deodorized and heat-treated, are no longer whole foods. They are not able to maintain healthy, functioning bodies, as we'll see later on in the book.

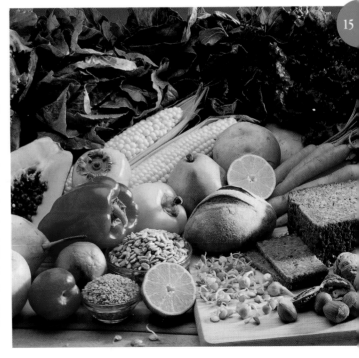

Eating whole food means eating food in its natural state–not processed or packaged.

15

Whole Food	Not Whole Food
• 100% whole wheat	• White flour
• Aged apple-cider vinegar	• Unaged (chemically produced) cider vinegar
• Brown rice	• White Rice
• Butter	• Margarine
• Carrot with skin	• Peeled carrot
• Evaporated sugarcane juice	• White sugar
• Nutrients from natural sources	• Nutrients from chemical sources*
• Potato with skin	• Peeled potato
• Pure maple syrup	• Maple-flavored sugar-based syrup, corn syrup
• Pure vanilla extract	• Synthetic vanilla extract
• Rapunzel® organic bouillon	• Bouillon with monosodium glutamate
• Sucanat® or Radapura®	• High-fructose corn syrup
• Whole apple	• Apple juice
• Whole barley	• Pearl barley
• Whole-grain cereal	• Cream of wheat cereal
• Whole-grain pasta	• White pasta

*There are many whole-food sources of nutrients such as calcium, magnesium and B vitamins. There are also supplements made from whole-food sources; they are labeled as such. You will find them in your health food store. Supplements made from chemical compounds are not whole foods and are often incomplete.

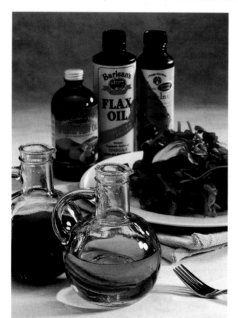

Whole-Food Fats and Oils

A natural, whole-foods diet does *not* mean a fat-free diet, or even a low-fat diet. Fats are necessary for life, especially the essential fatty acids *linoleic acid* and *alpha-linolenic acid*. These are found in flax, sesame and sunflower seeds, and in natural yogurt, buttermilk, kefir, natural cheese, raw nuts and free-range eggs. Fats and oils also contain vitamins and "companion" nutrients such as lignans and lecithin. Processing and refining, including heating, removes these nutrients. To ensure that you use a "healthy oil" check the label and be sure it says "unrefined." Use a wide range of unrefined oils for salad dressings, dips and mayonnaise, such as flax seed, walnut, hazelnut and pumpkin seed oils.

A whole-foods diet *does not include* artificially hardened (hydrogenated) fats, such as shortening and most margarines. These fats contain disease-causing trans-fatty acids and are not heart-healthy as often touted by the industry who makes them.

> ### Trans-Fatty Acids—the Fats to Avoid!
> Hydrogenation is a heat-treatment process used to make liquid oils hard, stabilizing them to prevent rancidity. How? The process removes the bio-active substances that make the oils healthy, because it is these healthy substances that make the oil go rancid (like all natural food eventually does). Removing these substances stabilizes the oils and prevents them from becoming rancid. By adding a hydrogen molecule the liquid becomes hard. This long-lasting product (along with promises of health and "low fat") sounds good to the consumer and is therefore an excellent marketing tool. What advertising and food labels don't convey, however, is that the heat process of hydrogenation converts good fatty acids (*cis-fatty* acids) into harmful fatty acids (*trans-fatty* acids).
>
> Food manufacturers tell us that trans-fatty acids behave like saturated fats, but in reality they are plastics, which the body cannot metabolize. Trans-fatty acids behave much differently in the human body than cis-fatty acids do. Instead of acting like a spark plug for fat metabolism, trans-fatty acids act more like an ill-fitting ignition key, unable to generate the spark that ignites fat metabolism. Worse, just as that ill-fitting key actually can break off and plug up the system, trans-fatty acids can plug up the liver, preventing the cis-fatty acids your body has absorbed from healthy food sources from performing properly.
> —*Good Fats and Oils*, by Siegfried Gursche
>   (*alive* Health Guide #17, 2000)

Margarine vs. Butter

Foods that have additives or preservatives, or have been altered, are not part of a whole-foods diet. Margarine is a synthetic food that is engineered from denatured ingredients that have been altered and so is not a whole or natural food. Hydrogenated margarine and foods like it are credited with causing free-radical damage, which can lead to atherosclerosis (hardening of the arteries).

Butter is a whole food. It is naturally solid at room temperature without adding anything to it. If you're concerned that butter is as bad for you as other animal fats, note that there is a

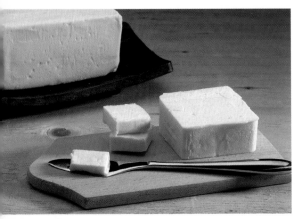

Butter is a whole food, margarine is not.

difference. Butter is not body fat, like the fat on a steak, it is a secreted fat, and contains a full spectrum of different types of healthy fatty acids and nutrients.

There's an expression that I use as a guideline for telling me if a food is a whole food: If God made it, eat it. If people made it, leave it alone. I conclude that God made butter and people made margarine. Eat butter and leave margarine alone.

Olive Oil–a Good Fat!

Olive oil is an essential part of a healthy diet and is ideal to cook with. The bitter principle (called oleuropein) in olives, olive oil and olive leaves has antiviral, antibacterial and antiprotozoic properties. This makes it a really healthy food. If you eat olives and olive oil on a regular basis, you are helping protect yourself from all kinds of illnesses and helping rid your body of some nasty things such as viruses, bacteria and parasites that might be hanging around in your system. Use olive oil for cooking, but keep the temperature below 220°F (106°C) to preserve its nutritional value.

Olive can be compared to wine. There are the cheap grades and the most expensive estate bottled varieties. When purchasing olive oil always look for "extra virgin." It is more expensive, however, you will find the best quality and taste in this grade.

Genetically Modified vs. Organic Foods

Genetically modified or genetically engineered foods are not proven to be safe. They are intended to grow and sell more produce, therefore generating more profit.

The only safe foods, as far as I am concerned, are labeled "certified organic" or "organically grown." This is especially true of all soybean products, including tofu, soya milk, miso, tamari and shoyu. My advice is please do not eat them unless they are organically grown and fermented. This will ensure that you are not eating pesticides, herbicides or genetically modified organisms.

I have always said that there are foods made for selling and foods made for eating. The foods made for selling last a long time on the shelf, do not get damaged if banged around a little and often can be stripped of the outer portions as they go bad

Do not eat soybean products unless they are organically grown and fermented. This will ensure that you are not eating pesticides, herbicides or genetically modified organisms.

(iceberg lettuce, for example). Real, whole food is made for eating. It has all the nutrients that are supposed to be in the food. It has to be handled carefully or it will go "off." It needs to be taken care of in the harvesting, shipping and storing. This is vital, living food.

Whole Foods Create Health . . . .

Whole foods will help you not only live longer, but live better. The foods that are healthy for your body are the foods that create health. If you eat a whole-foods diet, you reduce your chances of developing many of the degenerative diseases so common to seniors. This type of diet will also help you lose weight if you need to, and that in turn will help reduce your chances of developing over-weight-related conditions such as cardiovascular disease.

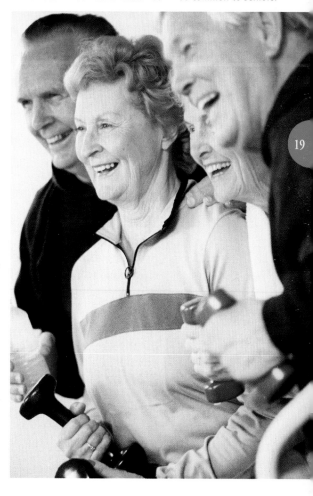

If you eat a whole-foods diet, you reduce your chances of developing many of the degenerative diseases so common to seniors.

19

Whole foods do not contain the manufactured, refined and heat-damaged fats, which means less chance of developing hardening of the arteries, diabetes, heart disease and some forms of cancer. Not only will your life expectancy increase, but your quality of life as well.

The high nutritional value of whole foods means that they can help prevent conditions related to deficiencies of specific vitamins or minerals. Whole foods will also save you from the refined, iodized table salt that creates kidney and blood pressure problems. Natural, unre-fined rock salt and sundried sea salt are healthy, as long as the daily intake remains below 6 to 7 grams, which is a heaping teaspoon.

B Vitamins are a Must!

B vitamin deficiencies are responsible for irritable bowel syndrome, nervous disorders, heart disease, depression, schizophrenia, dry skin and even dandruff. B vitamins help give your body energy by helping your body convert the carbohydrates (starch) to blood sugar, or glucose. Glucose is the fuel that runs your body. B vitamins also help your body to metabolize fats and protein. Your nervous system is also heavily dependent on B vitamins to stay healthy. Now you can see what eating white rice or white flour with the B vitamins removed can do to you! Brewer's yeast and other nutritional yeasts contain B vitamins and eating them is one way to supplement your Bs. A complete B vitamin supplement contains B_1, B_2, B_3, B_5, B_6, B_{12}, choline, inositol, p-aminobenzoic acid (PABA) and folic acid. The B family of vitamins must work together in a balance, so if you are purchasing a supplement from a health store be sure to get a B-complex.

Dark-green leafy vegetables contain chlorophyll, beta-carotene, the carotenoid xanthophyll, minerals such as calcium and magnesium, and B and C vitamins. The xanthophylls, along with vitamin E and the essential fatty acids, are useful in preventing and reversing age-related macular degeneration. Whole wheat is a major source of vitamin E. The germ of the wheat contains the majority of the vitamin E, and it is inside the starchy part of the wheat kernel, where it is protected from deterioration. The carotenoids and vitamin E are antioxidants that prevent oxidative damage in your body, according to research carried out at the Oakland University Eye Research Institute in Rochester, Michigan.

Fabulous Fiber

Whole foods contain more fiber, no question. Fiber in your diet improves your digestion in several ways. First, you have to chew fibrous foods more to break the fiber down. This is good because chewing starts digestion, especially of starches such as grains, potatoes, beans, corn, fruit and cereals. This is especially important after age forty-five, when digestion starts to slow down. Stress can slow down or stop digestion, so chewing is essential if you are stressed.

Second, fiber gives your intestines something to work on and this improves the muscles in your digestive tract. A high-fiber diet is to your intestines what sit-ups are to your tummy muscles: fiber tones up those muscles and helps them work more efficiently. This will help improve your digestion.

Third, fiber acts like a broom, sweeping stale fecal matter out of your intestines. Putrefying fecal matter can encourage many intestinal problems, including constipation, bad breath, diverticula (pouches created by herniation of the lining of the intestine) or even diverticulitis (an infection or abscess in a diverticulum).

The fiber sweeps stale matter out of your body, cleaning you out and allowing your intestines to function more efficiently. If stale feces remain in the intestines for too long, the risk for cancer, expecially colon cancer, increases many fold.

Fiber detoxifies. Sluggish digestion can encourage aging by slowing down the rate at which toxins and fecal matter leave your body. The longer they stay in your body, the more chance you have of reabsorbing the very poisons your body is working to get rid of through normal elimination. Your body will become exhausted trying to deal with these toxins and that will make you look and feel older. Fiber increases your bowel movements. Ensure that you have "to go" daily. Anything less than daily is constipation that needs to be dealt with. For more information read *Good Digestion* by Ken Babal (*alive* Natural Health Guide #25, 2000).

High-fiber whole food is detoxifying and improves digestion.

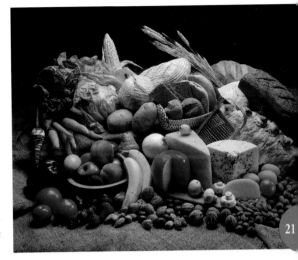

21

Enzymes

Another important element of the whole-foods way of eating is consuming your food raw. One suggestion is that 60 to 85 percent of your food should be eaten raw. If you eat lots of fruit, vegetables and sprouts, this is easy. The reason for this is that raw foods contain enzymes that help with the detoxification work carried out by your colon, kidneys, lungs and skin, in addition to aiding digestion. I generally put a garnish of chopped, fresh parsley and sprouts on all cooked foods.

Enzymes are the spark plugs of life! Without them, efficient nutrient absorption is impossible. Unsuspecting consumers do not realize that their refined, packaged and processed foods are devoid of enzymes. Enzyme-deficient, processed foods not only inhibit proper digestion; they tax the body's ability to function at an optimal level. Without enzymes all metabolic functions slow down, making the body more susceptible to disease.

By adding fresh enzyme-rich fruits and vegetables to our diets, eating fermented foods such as sauerkraut and yogurt and possibly supplementing the diet with digestive enzymes, we can look better, feel better and maintain health. Remember to chew your food well, which stimulates the natural enzymes in the body to start working.

All-Important Antioxidants

Free-radical damage contributes to aging. Even if we are careful about what we eat, we are bombarded by free radicals from the environment. But the good news is that you can reduce free-radical damage by increasing your intake of antioxidants. Whole foods are best for this because they contain a wide, balanced range of antioxidants and other nutrients. In 1994, an article in the *Journal of the American Medical Association* recommended certain antioxidants every day to prevent chronic, age-related diseases:

- 250-1000 milligrams of vitamin C
- 100-400 International Units of vitamin E
- 10-30 milligrams of beta carotene (vitamin A)

Other important antioxidants are the minerals selenium, manganese, zinc, copper and sulfur; the amino acids cysteine, methionine, glutathionine and taurine; bioflavonoids; coenzyme Q10; and vitamins B_2, B_3 and K. A diverse, whole-foods diet is the best way to obtain these nutrients.

Avoid Aluminum!

Aluminum enters our bodies through food, water, antiperspirants, antacids and some cooking utensils. This relates to a theory of aging known as "cross-linking," when the binding together of proteins, carbohydrates, abnormal cells and other substances with the assistance of an agent such as aluminum. These substances make tight knots that just keep getting bigger and more tangled. They collect in our bones, contributing to osteoporosis, and in our brains, causing Alzheimer's disease. You can help reduce this process by replacing your aluminum cookware, by not using antiperspirants containing aluminum and by not taking antacids. Equally important is a natural, whole-foods diet, which will slow the rate of cross-linking and break down the "tangles."

How to Embrace a Whole Foods Diet . . . .

When you change to a whole-food diet, start gradually. You might be increasing the fiber in your diet by a little or a lot. Adding fiber can cause changes in your digestive system, so it is best to go slowly and do not tax your system. If you find that adding fiber and whole foods to your diet gives you gas or intestinal distress, chew each mouthful until it's liquid so that your digestion improves. This is important, because good digestion is the key to feeling young. It won't take long before your body is used to the increased fiber and you'll be rewarded with boundless energy.

If this kind of chewing helps only slightly, then you might need to take digestive enzymes. As you age, your digestion, like other parts of your body, starts to slow down. The most comprehensive kind of digestive aid contains enzymes that digest all kinds of foods. A good supplement will contain protease, amylase, lipase, cellulase, sucrase, lactase, maltase, alpha galactosidase and bromelain. Health food stores carry a wide variety of digestive enzymes. Ask for advice.

Eating whole food is fun, healthful and rewarding.

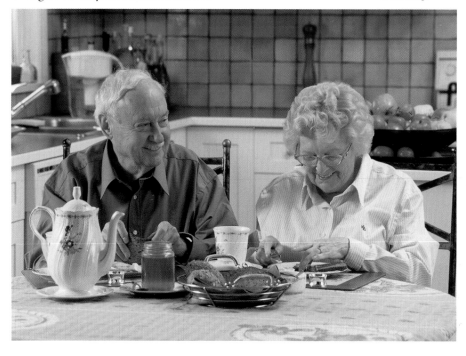

Another strategy is to eat more often, but eat less at each meal. Try five or six small meals each day instead of the usual three. Always include one item of raw food: an apple, tomato, carrot or celery sticks, radishes, green lettuce, coleslaw, or whatever you can lay your hands on. Melons, pineapples and grapes are excellent. This way, your body will have enough enzymes to break down your food and therefore make use of all the nutrients your whole food is providing. Eating too much overloads your digestive system so that it can't assimilate food. An additional benefit of eating less: studies have shown that people who eat less live longer. And research on rats has shown that the benefits of eating less can be obtained even if this strategy is adopted in mid-life. It's not too late!

Use as many organic ingredients as you can find. Sprayed grains, fruits and vegetables tax the immune system. If you cannot find organic food, remember to wash all fruits, vegetables and grains before you eat or cook them. Most health food stores carry a produce-washing product.

Whole Foods Transition	
• start gradually	• eat less
• chew food well	• eat raw food
• eat more frequently	• buy organic whenever possible

What Else Should I Do?

Once, when I was teaching vegetarian cooking in Toronto, I wiped off a fresh mushroom before cooking it and one of my students asked why I wasn't peeling it. She had come from Europe where, apparently, the skins from mushrooms gathered in the wild were too tough and dirty to eat, and she had continued her practice of peeling mushrooms when she came to Canada. In North America, where mushrooms are cultivated, we just brush, wipe or rinse mushrooms. If the skin of a food is edible, then you should eat it. If the skin is not edible, then don't consider eating it. You should eat the skin of apples, pears, peaches, grapes and green beans, but don't think that you have to eat the skins of cantaloupe, watermelon, bananas or pea pods!

Examine all your food habits. You might have habits that you got from your neighbor, your school, or your parents that no longer serve you. Look into why and how you treat your food to see if there are habits that you have adopted that contribute to eating fractionated foods.

Convert Your Own Recipes

When you start to eat whole foods you can convert many of your favorite recipes to whole-foods recipes. Once your taste buds enjoy whole foods in your favorite recipes, you can venture into uncharted waters and try new recipes. Of course, I hope you'll try some of my favorite whole-food recipes, which are featured in this book.

If the Recipe Calls For:	Substitute With:
Bread flour	100% whole-wheat bread flour*
Liquid oil	Extra-virgin olive oil
Molasses	Organic Sucanat® blackstrap unsulfured molasses
Pastry flour	Whole-wheat pastry flour*
Prepared salad dressing	Make your own from fresh ingredients
Regular white pasta	Whole-grain pasta
Salt	Natural sea salt
Shortening or margarine	Butter
White or brown sugar	Sucanat® or Rapadura®
White rice	Brown rice* (brown rice takes longer to cook)
White vinegar	Natural apple cider vinegar

*Many people start slowly by replacing half the white flour or rice products with whole-grain flours or rice. This will be a gradual change that your family might not even notice. You can change to total whole-grain products once you have become accustomed to them.

Just as the proof of the pudding is in the eating, so it will be with your venture into whole foods. When you start to feel more alert, more alive, younger and less sick, you will begin to love whole foods. Everyone that I have known who has changed to a whole-food diet has been glad they did. You will be, too. If you can change your diet and stick to it for a few months, you'll be a convert to whole foods forever. Feel better and live longer!

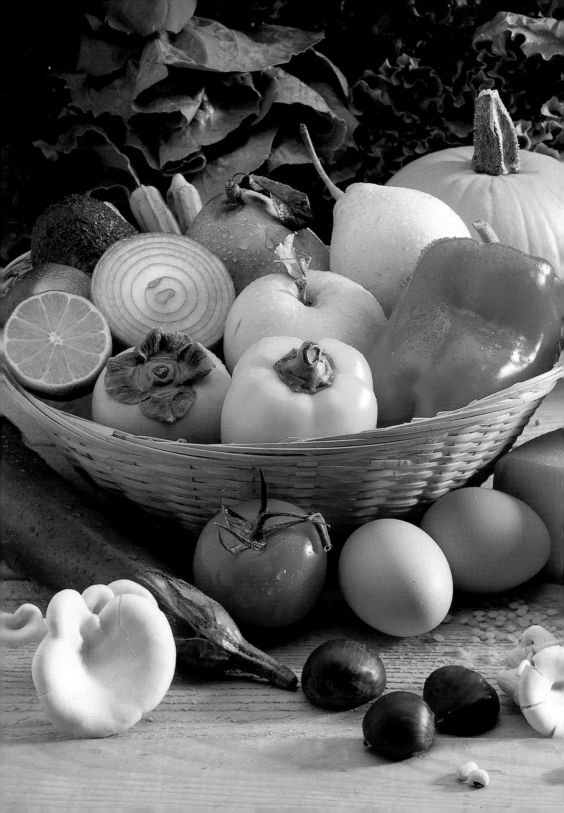

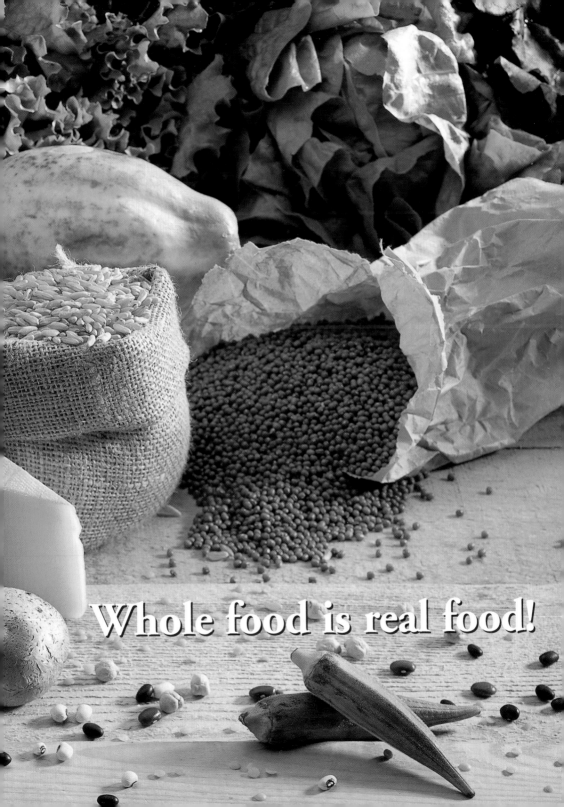

Whole food is real food!

Whole-Foods Breakfast

The ideal whole-foods breakfast starts with whole-grain cereals and breads. Adding nuts and fruit enhances your essential fatty acid, vitamin and mineral intake. You can eat this meal any time of the day, don't be stuck in the "I must have cold cereal for breakfast" routine.

2 cups (500 ml) **millet puffs**

¼ cup (60 ml) **water chestnuts, roasted and sliced**

¼ cup (60 ml) **nuts of your choice**

½ cup (125 ml) **mixed dried fruit, such as raisins and apricots**

Combine cereal, nuts and dried fruit in bowls. Serve with eggs, whole grain toast, whole milk and freshly squeezed juice.

Serves 2

walnut

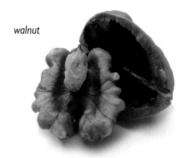

Roasted Chestnuts
Look for fresh chestnuts in the shell and prepare them yourself. Rich and nutty when roasted, chestnuts are low in fat, which makes them easy to digest.

Preheat oven to 375°F (190°C). With the tip of a knife cut a small cross on each chestnut shell. Place in a baking dish and bake in the oven for 15 to 20 minutes. The chestnut is done when the cut skin curls up. (Or roast in a skillet on top of the stove.) Break the skin and scoop out the chestnut flesh using a spoon.

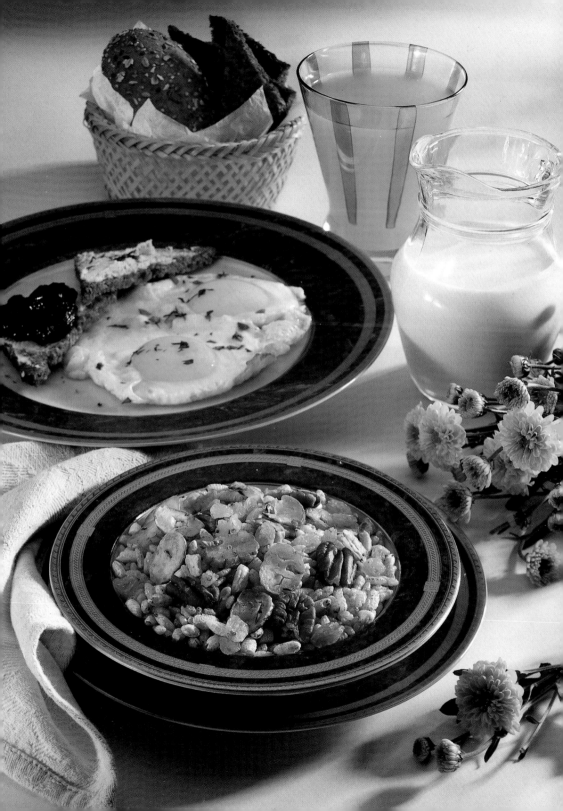

Raw Vegetable Snack

It's important to eat raw food every day to obtain the enzymes that are essential to life and health. As we age, the body has less ability to manufacture its own enzymes. Eating foods that contains enzymes saves the body's energy from having to make enzymes. In addition, use as many organic ingredients as you can find; your immune system will be less taxed when you use unsprayed grains, fruits and vegetables.

Baby carrots

Asparagus

Jicama root, cut in sticks

Celery, cut in sticks

Romaine lettuce

Broccoli florets

Cauliflower florets

Serve vegetables with yogurt-mint dressing or a simple quark-flax seed oil dip.

Yogurt-Mint Dressing

½ tsp dried yellow mustard seed
½ tsp dried black mustard, caraway and
   coriander seed
½ cup (125 ml) natural yogurt or kefir
2 tbsp cold-pressed walnut oil or flax seed oil
1 tbsp fresh lemon or lime juice
1 tbsp fresh mint, chopped
Vegetable salt (such as Herbamare), to taste

In a small saucepan, heat spices on low heat for 4 to 5 minutes (no longer, otherwise the spices will turn bitter). In a coffee grinder, grind spices into a powder. In a bowl, whisk together yogurt, oil, lemon juice, mint, salt and pepper, and spices.

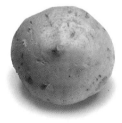

jicama

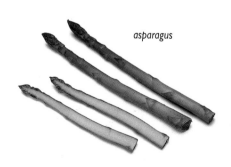

asparagus

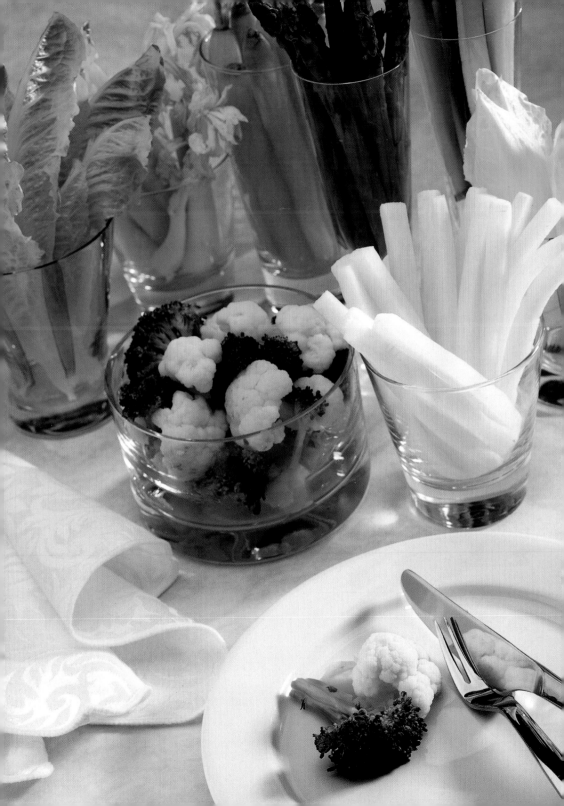

Heart of Romaine
Salad with Apple and Walnut

As we age, we require more antioxidants. Living in polluted environments increases this need as well. Tender and succulent, the heart of Romaine, like most green leafy vegetables, provides you with antioxidants to inhibit free-radical damage as well as carotenoids, useful in preventing macular degeneration.

1 heart of Romaine, cut in half

1 Granny Smith apple, cored and sliced

½ cup (125 ml) **walnuts, toasted**

¾ cup (200 g) **blue cheese, crumbled**

Dressing:

¼ cup (60 ml) **grainy mustard**

3 tbsp unrefined walnut or flax seed oil

2 tbsp honey

1 tsp fresh lemon juice

1 tsp shallot, minced

½ tsp garlic, minced

In a bowl, whisk together dressing ingredients until emulsified. Place romaine onto plates, arrange apple on top and sprinkle with walnuts and blue cheese. Drizzle dressing over top and serve.

Serves 2

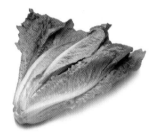

Romaine lettuce

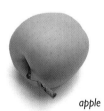

apple

Remember to avoid supermarket dressings as they contain harmful trans fats. Prepare your own from fresh, wholesome ingredients, the most important of which are unrefined oils that are flavorful and rich in linoleic and alpha-linolenic essential fatty acids.

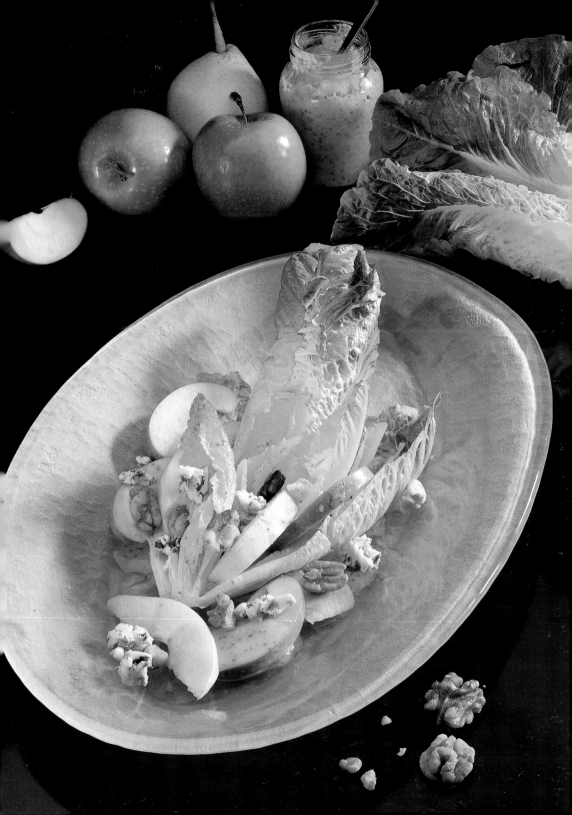

Green Bean Salad
with Panroasted Belgian Endive

Antioxidants, fresh air, sunlight and exercise together slow the aging process. Eating a whole-foods diet is the best way to obtain a balance of antioxidants to fight the free-radical damage that contributes to aging.

2 cups (500 ml) **green beans, cut 3"** (8 cm)

2 Belgian endives, cut in half

1 tbsp extra-virgin olive oil

1 cup (250 ml) **red onion, sliced**

½ cup (125 ml) **feta cheese, crumbled**

Classic Vinaigrette:

4 tbsp extra-virgin olive oil

1 tbsp white wine vinegar

1 medium shallot, minced

½ tsp garlic, minced

1 tsp fresh herbs of your choice, chopped

3 ½ tsp fresh lemon juice

1 tsp Dijon mustard

Sea salt and fresh ground pepper, to taste

1-2 drops unpasteurized honey (optional)

Blanch beans in a pot of boiling salted water for 4 to 5 minutes. Drain and rinse with cold water.

In the meantime, panroast Belgian endive in oil until both sides are golden brown.

In a bowl, whisk together all dressing ingredients. Place beans and onion in a bowl and toss with the dressing. Place salad onto plates, arrange endive around and crumble feta cheese on top.

Serves 2

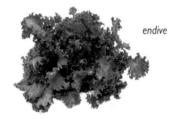

endive

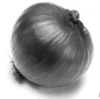

red onion

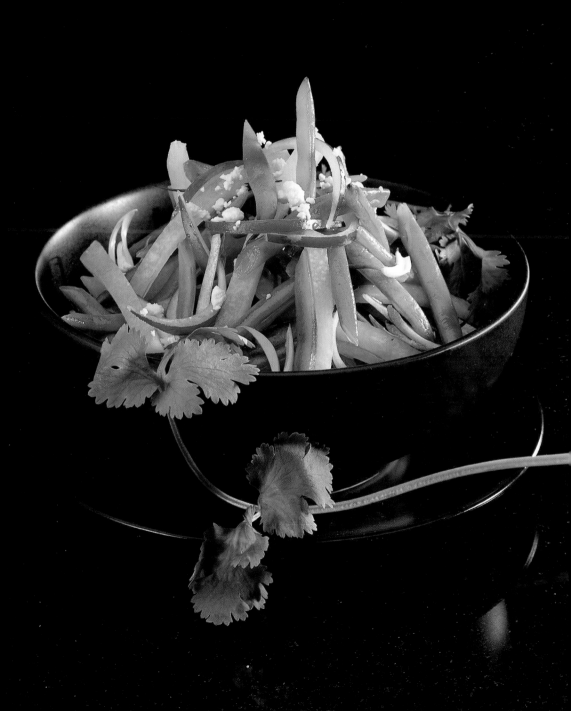

Mixed Greens with
Herb Croutons and Swiss Emmenthal

The whole-foods kitchen always includes fresh herbs. Herbs not only delight the taste buds, they're rich in vitamins and minerals and provide many healing benefits. The croutons tossed in fresh herbs, provide fiber, vitamins A, C and iron, and aid in digestion and circulation.

2 cups (500 ml) **whole-grain bread, cubed**

1 tbsp butter

1 tbsp fresh mixed herbs (Italian parsley, thyme, oregano, basil, rosemary), **finely chopped**

2 cups (500 ml) **mixed organic greens**

1 cup (250 ml) **cherry tomatoes**

1 cup (250 ml) **Swiss Emmenthal cheese, cubed**

⅓ cup (85 ml) **Classic Vinaigrette** (page 34)

To make the croutons, melt butter in a pan and toss bread cubes until golden brown. Place croutons in a bowl, sprinkle with mixed herbs and toss well.

Place greens, tomato and cheese in a separate bowl and toss with the vinaigrette. Place salad onto plates, garnish with croutons and serve.

Serves 2

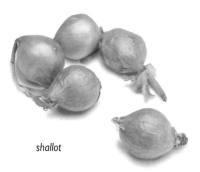

shallot

A quick and easy way to mix your vinaigrette is to place all the ingredients in a screw-top jar, cover and shake well. Place your vinaigrettes or dressings in a jar and store them for up to 2 weeks in the refrigerator.

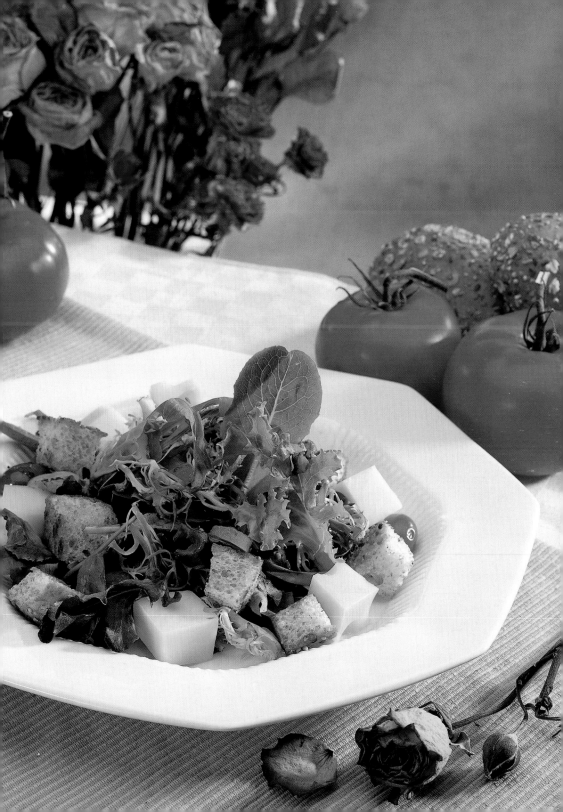

Croque Monsieur
(Grilled Cheese Sandwich)

The grilled cheese sandwich is a favorite at every age. The sandwich is like a chameleon, it goes with whatever the taste and time of day best suits you. It's especially good accompanied with fresh fruit or salad. Remember to use only real cheese that is natural and white; orange cheese is dyed and much of the cheese on the market is highly processed.

1 whole-wheat foccaccio, quartered

8 slices Swiss Emmenthal cheese, thinly sliced

2 tbsp + 1 tbsp butter, at room temperature

2 tbsp extra-virgin olive oil

2 eggs, beaten

Pinch sea salt

Pinch cinnamon

Organic maple syrup

Spread butter onto each foccaccio slice then place cheese in between two slices. Cut the crust from the edges, then cut diagonally. Beat eggs in a bowl and add a pinch of salt and cinnamon. Dip foccaccio in egg batter. Heat butter and olive oil in a pan and fry foccaccio pieces until both sides are golden brown. Serve with maple syrup and fresh salad or fruit.

Serves 2

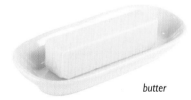

butter

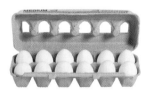

free-range eggs

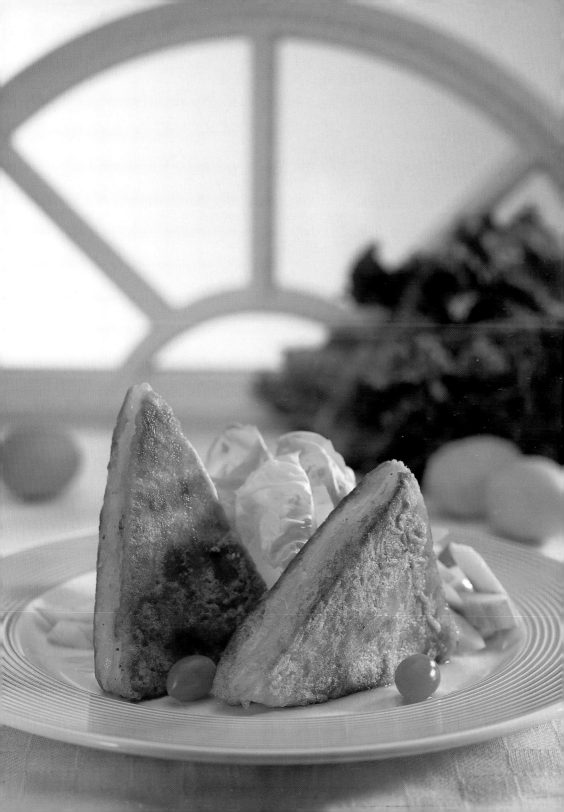

Simple Steamed Vegetables

A meal doesn't need to be fancy to be flavorful and healthy. Enjoy the tastes of these simple vegetables with a hearty whole-grain bread and obtain the fiber needed to aid digestion and detoxify.

6–8 baby carrots, peeled

6–8 small parsnips, peeled

2 yams, peeled and cut in strips

2 small kohlrabi, peeled

4 small beets, peeled

2 tbsp butter

Steam carrots, parsnip and yam for 5 minutes, kohlrabi separately for 7 to 10 minutes and beets separately for 25 to 30 minutes. Melt butter, drizzle over top the vegetables and serve.

Serves 2

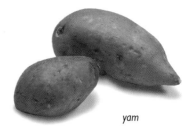

yam

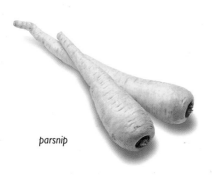

parsnip

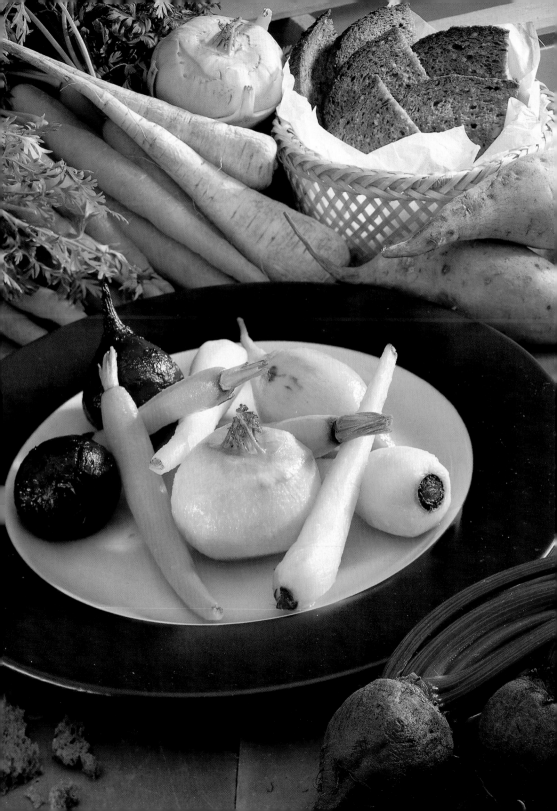

All-in-One Potato Meal

When enjoying this all-in-one meal you won't know where all the subtle flavors are coming from, just that it's an incredibly delicious combination of simple wholesome ingredients. Significant amounts of minerals are found underneath the potato's skin so don't peel them or you'll lose important nutrients and fiber.

2 lbs (1 kg) **red nugget potatoes, cut in half**

4 cloves garlic, peeled

4 tbsp extra-virgin olive oil, divided

1 cup (250 ml) **leek, sliced** **¼"** (5 mm)

1 tbsp fresh rosemary, chopped

1 tsp caraway seeds

Vegetable salt (such as Herbamare)**, to taste**

1 cup (250 ml) **feta cheese, crumbled**

Place garlic cloves in a small ovenproof bowl with 1 tablespoon of olive oil and bake in the oven at 375°F (190°C) for 15 minutes.

In the meantime, cook potato in a large pot of boiling salted water for 10 to 12 minutes or until tender yet firm. Drain and place in a large bowl.

Sauté leek and rosemary in 1 tablespoon of oil for 3 minutes until soft then add to potato; mix well. Add roasted garlic, 2 tablespoons of oil, caraway seeds and Herbamare; mix again. Place potato mixture onto plates, crumble feta cheese over top and serve.

Serves 2

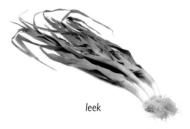

leek

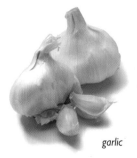

garlic

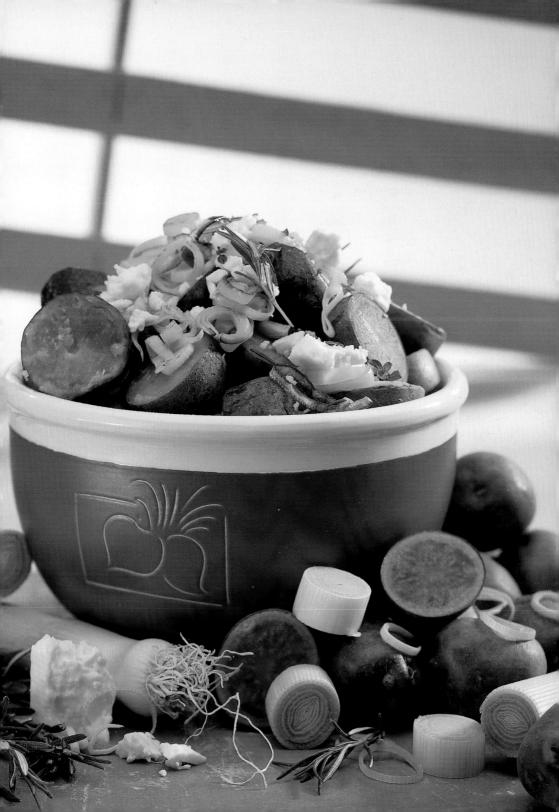

Pear-Corn Chowder

Soft and sweet, the pear in this unique chowder recipe literally melts in your mouth and is complemented by the crunchy texture of fresh corn. Pears contain vitamin A and phosphorus and according to Chinese medicine, energize the stomach and lungs.

2 cups (500 ml) **fresh corn kernels**

1 cup (250 ml) **celery, diced**

1 cup (250 ml) **onion, diced**

2 tbsp extra-virgin olive oil

1 cup (125 ml) **cream**

2 cups (500 ml) **vegetable stock**

2 pears, peeled and diced

1 tsp caraway or coriander seeds

Vegetable salt (such as Herbamare)**, to taste**

1 tbsp butter

Sauté corn, celery and onion in oil until soft then add vegetable stock and cream and cook for 10 minutes. Add pear, caraway (or coriander), salt and pepper; cook for 3 minutes longer. Stir in butter and serve.

Serves 2

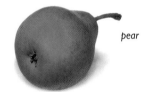

pear

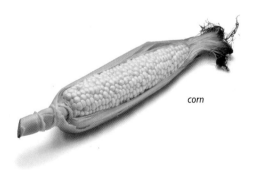

corn

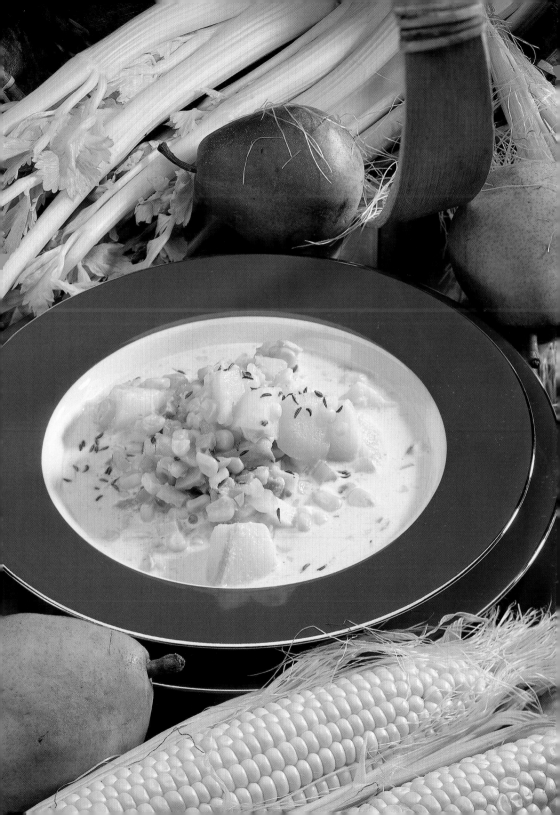

Tomato Stuffed
with Vegetable-Rice Confetti

This colorful and hearty dish is sure to please the eyes and palates of your whole-food-loving guests. The versatile tomato, already rich in vitamins A, B-complex and C, potassium and phosphorus is stuffed with many more nutrients such as iron, vitamin E, protein and linoleic acid from the brown rice.

2 large tomatoes

1 tbsp butter

1 tbsp + 1 tbsp extra-virgin olive oil

2 cloves garlic, minced

½ cup (125 mL) **onion, diced**

½ cup (125 mL) **carrot, diced**

½ cup (125 mL) **celery, diced**

½ cup (125 mL) **yellow or red bell pepper, diced**

½ cup (125 mL) **fresh corn kernels**

1 tbsp fresh rosemary, chopped

1 cup (250 mL) **cooked brown rice**

Vegetable salt (such as Herbamare)**, to taste**

Sauce:

1 shallot, minced

1 clove garlic, minced

1 tbsp butter

¼ cup (60 mL) **vegetable stock**

1 tbsp fresh tarragon, chopped

1 tbsp fresh lemon juice

1 cup (250 mL) **whip cream**

Preheat the oven to 375°F (190°C).

Cut the top ½" (1 cm) off the tomatoes and scoop out the inside flesh, making a cup. Dice the flesh and set aside.

Heat butter and oil in a large pan on medium and sauté diced tomato, garlic, onion, carrot, celery, bell pepper and corn until soft. Add rosemary and rice; mix thoroughly. Stuff the tomato cups with the vegetable-rice mixture then season with salt and pepper and brush with olive oil. Bake in the oven for 15 minutes.

To make the sauce, gently sauté shallot and garlic in butter until soft. Add vegetable stock, tarragon, lemon juice and cream then reduce by one-third. Pour sauce onto plates, place stuffed tomato on top and serve.

Serves 2

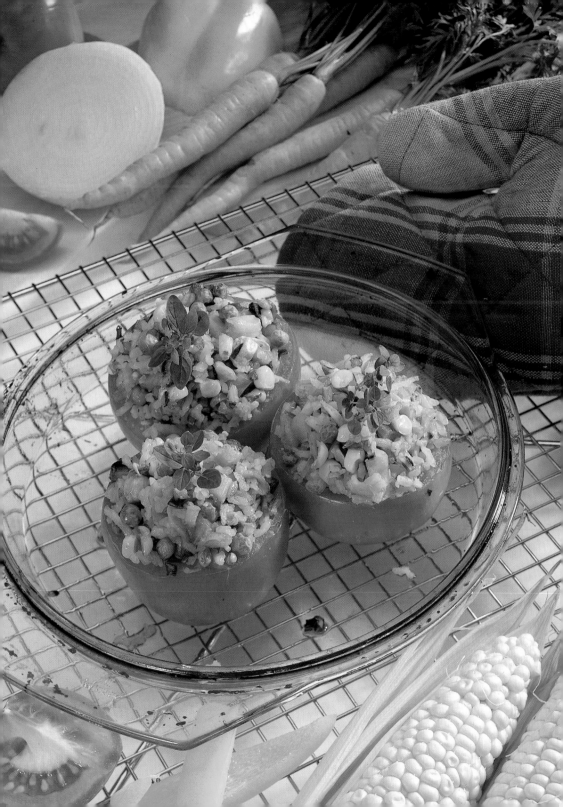

Zucchini-Tomato
Gratin with Herb-Cheese Buns

The tomatoes in this sumptuous gratin are an excellent ingredient for all ages. Recent studies demonstrate that tomato-lovers live longer and have reduced incidences of prostate, breast and digestive-tract cancers.

Buns:

1 cup (250 ml) **whole-grain bread flour**

½ cup (125 ml) **whole-wheat flour**

1 tbsp baking powder

½ tbsp evaporated cane juice or Rapadura

1 ½ cups (375 ml) **Gruyère or aged Cheddar cheese, grated**

1 tsp fresh Italian parsley, finely chopped

2 egg whites

2 tbsp extra-virgin olive oil

¾ cups (180 ml) **whole milk**

1 tbsp rolled oats

Gratin:

3 large vine-ripened tomatoes, sliced ¼" (5 mm) **thick**

2 large zucchinis, sliced ¼" (5 mm) **thick**

Herbamare, to taste

Juice of ½ lime

3 tbsp extra-virgin olive oil

1 tbsp fresh herbs of your choice, such as oregano, basil or marjoram

½ cup (125 ml) **Parmesan, Pecorino or Asiago cheese, freshly grated**

1 tbsp butter, to grease pan

Preheat oven 375°F (190°C). Grease a 10" (25 cm) round baking dish and large muffin cups with butter.

Gratin: Arrange tomato and zucchini in the baking dish, season with Herbamare and drizzle with lime juice and olive oil. Bake for 10 minutes then remove from oven and sprinkle with herbs then cheese. Grill under the broiler for 5 minutes until the cheese melts.

Buns: Combine flours, baking powder and Rapadura in a large bowl. Stir in cheese and herbs. In a separate bowl, combine egg whites, oil and milk then add to the dry ingredients, stirring until just moistened. Fill muffin cups three-quarters full then sprinkle oats on top and bake for 25 to 30 minutes.

Serves 2

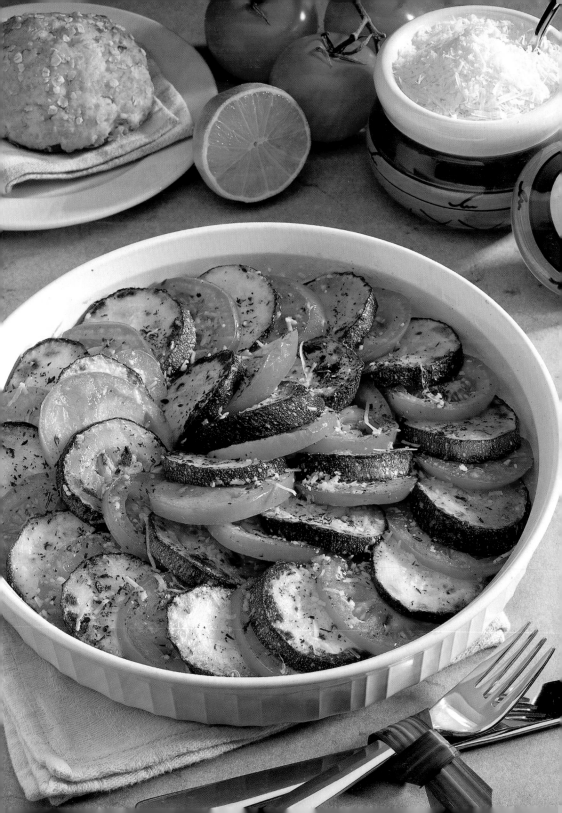

Pasta Verde

Older people tend to lack vitamins B6, B12, folic acid and calcium. This combination of rich green vegetables supplies vitamins A, B-complex, C and E, and calcium, iron and potassium. Together with the whole grain pasta, sunflower seeds and cheese, this is a whole-foods experience to enjoy time and time again.

7 oz (200 g) **whole-wheat linguine**

½ cup (125 ml) **broccoli florets**

6–8 stalks asparagus tips, cut 3" (8 cm)

½ cup (125 ml) **snow peas**

½ cup (125 ml) **celery, diced**

½ cup (125 ml) **green onion, cut 3"** (8 cm)

2 cloves garlic, minced

1 tbsp butter

1 tbsp extra-virgin olive oil

1 tbsp fresh oregano, chopped

2 tbsp sunflower seeds

Parmesan cheese, shaved

Cook linguine in a pot of boiling salted water; drain, rinse with cold water and set aside.

Blanch vegetables in a pot of boiling salted water for 3 minutes. Drain and rinse under cold water.

Sauté garlic in butter and oil in a large pan until golden. Add vegetables and oregano; toss well. Add pasta, season with salt and pepper; toss again. Place pasta onto plates, sprinkle with sunflower seeds and Parmesan, and serve.

Serves 2

Whole-Grain Pasta

1 cup (250 ml) whole-wheat bread flour
1 cup (250 ml) barley flour
1 tsp sea salt
2 tbsp extra-virgin olive oil
2 organic eggs
A few drops of water, as needed

Food processor method: Sift flours and sea salt together into the bowl of a food processor. Add oil and eggs. Process until a soft ball forms. Add a few drops of water as needed to make the dough form. Do not add more than a tablespoon of water or it will be difficult to roll the pasta. If your flour has a lot of bran that is not ground up, it will dry out the dough so sift it out before measuring the flours.

Hand mixing method: Sift the dry ingredients onto a clean surface. Make a well in the center and put eggs and olive oil in it. Begin incorporating the flour into the center well mixing with a wooden spoon or fork, then use your hands. Knead it several times once thoroughly mixed. Generally when mixed by hand no water is needed.

Wrap in plastic and refrigerate for about 15 minutes. Remove from the refrigerator and let sit for another 5 minutes while you prepare the pasta machine. Keep the pasta covered while rolling it according to the directions for the pasta maker.

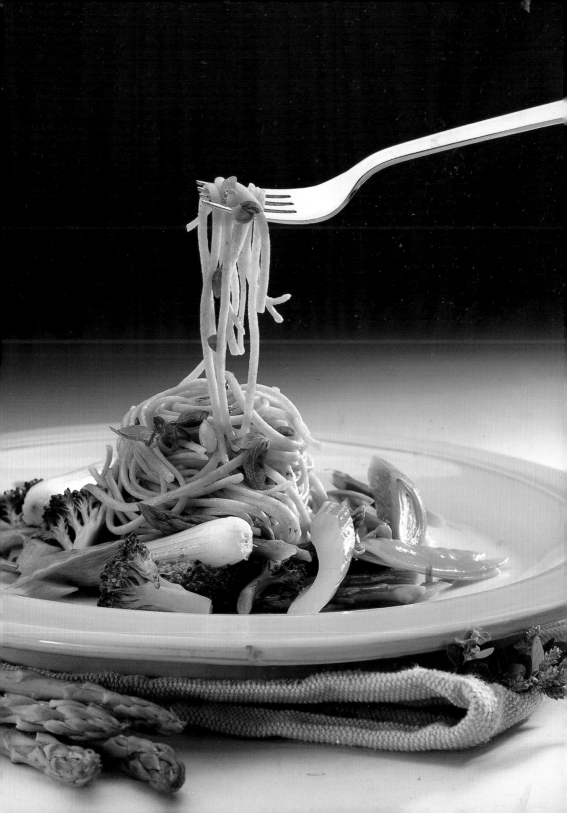

Cottage Cheese-
Vegetable Stuffed Pasta Shells

Pasta made with whole grains offer superior nutrition, containing the precious nutrients–protein, fiber, vitamins and minerals–that are concentrated in the outer membrane and germ of the grain. Adding parsley will balance the dairy fat in the cottage cheese and help you digest it better. In fact, parsley helps to improve the digestion of fats in most meals.

12 large whole-grain pasta shells

2 cloves garlic, minced

¼ **cup** (60 ml) **shallot or white onion, finely diced**

¼ **cup** (60 ml) **green onion, finely diced**

½ **cup** (60 ml) **red bell pepper, finely diced**

½ **cup** (60 ml) **yellow bell pepper, finely diced**

1 tbsp extra-virgin olive oil

1 tbsp fresh lemon juice

2 tbsp fresh Italian parsley, chopped

1 ½ cups (375 ml) **cottage cheese**

Vegetable salt (such as Herbamare)**, to taste**

Cook pasta shells in a pot of boiling salted water until al dente. Drain and set aside.

In a pan, sauté garlic, onions and peppers in oil until soft. Place sautéed vegetables in a bowl then add lemon juice and parsley; mix well. Add cottage cheese, season with salt and pepper; mix again.

Fill the pasta shells with the cottage cheese-vegetable mixture.

Serves 2

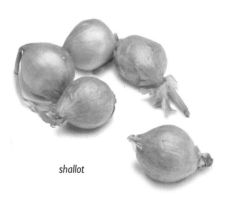

shallot

Serve with simple mixed greens and sprouts. Assimilation of nutrients decreases with age, therefore sprouts are beneficial because fats, proteins and starches have been broken down into easily digestible forms.

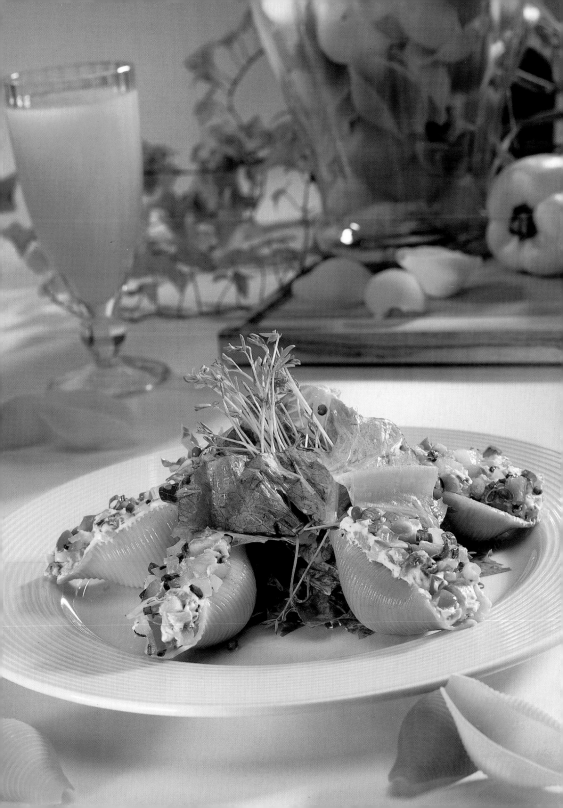

Marinated Portobello
Mushrooms with Vegetable Ratatouille

When you feel depleted of vitamins and minerals, this dish gives you nutrients from the ground and replenishes your body supply.

2 large Portobello mushrooms

2 tbsp + 1 tbsp extra-virgin olive oil

1 tbsp balsamic vinegar

2 Belgian endives, cut in half

Ratatouille:

1 cup (250 ml) **eggplant, cubed**

1 cup (250 ml) **zucchini, cubed**

½ cup (125 ml) **oven-dried tomatoes** (recipe below)

½ cup (125 ml) **bocconcini or buffalo mozzarella**

Marinade:

2 cloves garlic, sliced

1 tsp fresh cilantro, chopped

¼ **cup** (60 mL) **balsamic vinegar**

¼ **cup** (60 mL) **extra-virgin olive oil**

2 tsp fresh lemon juice

1 tsp fresh rosemary, chopped

Sea salt and fresh ground pepper or Herbamare, to taste

Pinch chili flakes

Thoroughly wipe clean the mushrooms with a paper towel and scrape out the inside black parts with a spoon. Don't wash the mushrooms as they will absorb water. (Don't throw out the stems, put them in a soup or pasta.)

In a bowl, whisk together marinade ingredients then add mushrooms, cover and let sit for 4 hours, turning every 2 hours. In the meantime, sauté eggplant and zucchini in oil for 5 to 7 minutes until soft. Add oven-dried tomatoes and bocconcini; toss well.

In a pan, grill Belgian endives in a bit of oil until golden on both sides. In another frying pan, heat oil over medium heat and fry the mushrooms, pressing them flat and turning once so that all surfaces are browned. Remove from heat and place onto plates. Drizzle with oil and balsamic vinegar, place eggplant-zucchini ratatouille and endive on top and serve.

Serves 2

Oven-dried Tomatoes
Cut 2 lbs (1 kg) of Roma tomatoes into small wedges, sprinkle with coarse sea salt and place in the oven at 200°F (190°C) for 4 to 5 hours. Remove from oven, cool then store in a jar with 2 tablespoons of olive oil and chopped fresh basil. Place in the refrigerator, where it will keep for up to two weeks.

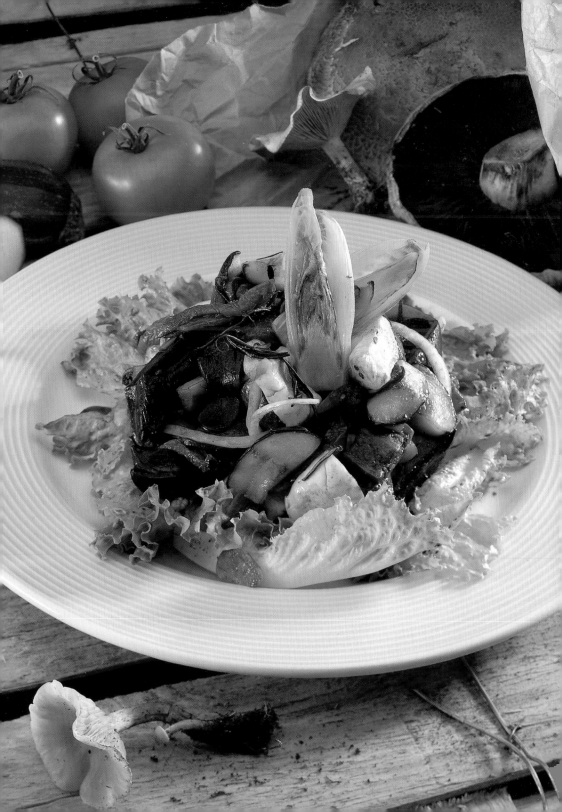

Curry Vegetable Stew

Vary the vegetables in this wholesome stew with whatever is in season. You can use fresh peas, summer squash, zucchini or pumpkin; the variations are unlimited. Ginger is excellent for improving digestion so include it in as many recipes as possible for taste and health.

1 cup (250 ml) **potato, cut in chunks**

1 cup (250 ml) **parsnip, cut in chunks**

1 cup (250 ml) **green beans, cut 3"** (8 cm)

1 cup (250 ml) **okra**

1 cup (250 ml) **tomatoes, cut in chunks**

1 cup (250 ml) **red onion, sliced**

4 cloves garlic

1 tsp ginger, minced

1 tsp curry powder

2 tbsp extra-virgin olive oil

1 cup (250 ml) **vegetable stock**

1 tbsp fresh rosemary, chopped

1 tsp coriander seed

Cook potato and parsnip in a pot of boiling water for 7 to 10 minutes until tender. Drain and set aside. Blanch beans and okra for 4 to 5 minutes then drain and rinse under cold water; set aside.

In a large pan, sauté garlic, ginger, vegetables and curry in oil for 2 to 3 minutes until soft. Add vegetable stock, rosemary and coriander; cover and simmer for 7 to 10 minutes. Serve with brown rice.

Serves 2

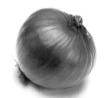

red onion

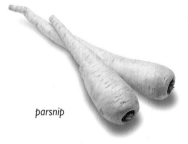

parsnip

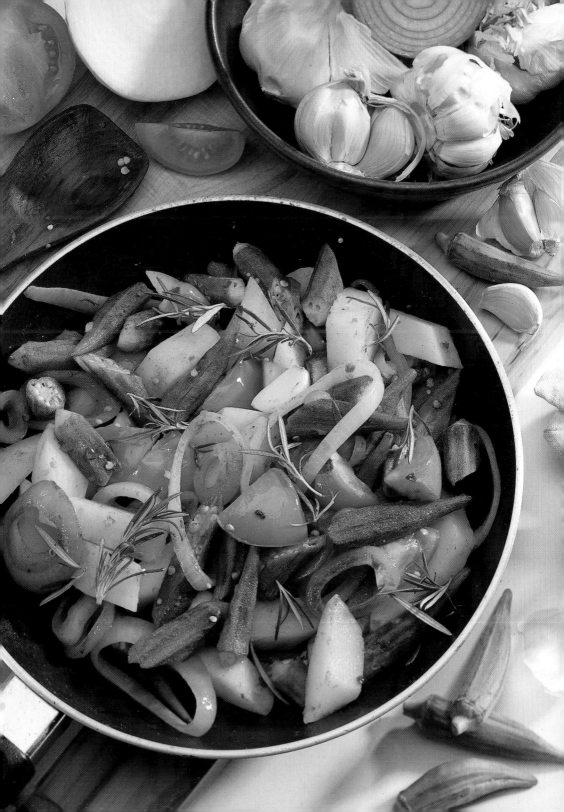

Vegetable-Tempeh
Stirfry with Crispy Rice Noodles

Variety in life keeps you going strong. I'm positive you'll enjoy the Asian flavors in this dish. Tempeh is a fermented soy food that's easily digested and a great source of vitamin B12. Studies show that eating soy lowers cholesterol levels and benefits the cardiovascular system. Look for organic tempeh grown from non-genetically altered soy beans.

1 bundle rice noodles

1 tbsp fresh cilantro, chopped

2 tbsp extra-virgin olive oil

2 tbsp toasted sesame seed oil

1 cup (250 ml) **snow peas**

1 cup (250 ml) **celery, sliced**

1 cup (250 ml) **carrot, sliced**

1 cup (250 ml) **onion, sliced**

1 cup (250 ml) **leek, chopped**

1 cup (250 ml) **okra**

1 cup (250 ml) **baby corn**

½ package tempeh, cubed

1 tsp ginger, minced

2 tbsp organic tamari or soy sauce

¼ cup (60 ml) **fresh coconut juice** (optional)

Place rice noodle in a bowl of hot (not boiling) water and soak for 10 minutes until soft. Drain noodles into a bowl and stir in cilantro. Heat olive oil in a pan on high then twist noodles around a fork and drop into the oil, pressing down with the fork to form a 5" (8 cm) patty. Panfry each side for 4 to 5 minutes until golden brown.

In the meantime, heat sesame oil over medium heat and sauté vegetables, tempeh, ginger, tamari and coconut juice for 5 to 7 minutes until soft.

Arrange rice patties onto plates, place stirfried vegetables on top and serve.

Serves 2

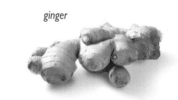

ginger

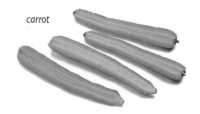

carrot

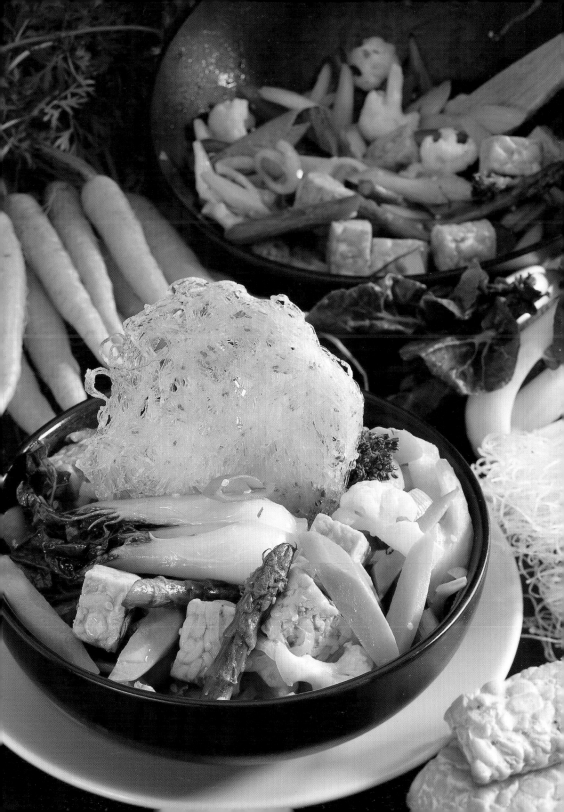

Apple Pie

The apples stay fresh-tasting and crisp in this whole-food version of a classic. Go ahead and indulge–this pie is full of wholesome ingredients. Apples are easy to digest and rich in fiber and minerals; freshly shelled walnuts and pecans are excellent sources of essential fats.

Pastry:

1 ½ cups (375 ml) **whole-wheat flour**

Pinch sea salt

1 free-range egg yolk

2 tbsp + 2 tbsp butter, at room temperature

2 tbsp natural milk or water, cold

2 tbsp natural sugar such as Rapadura

2 cups (500 ml) **uncooked chickpeas, beans or rice, for blind baking**

Filling:

8 medium-size Granny Smith apples

2 tbsp maple syrup

1 tbsp butter

½ cup (125 ml) **sultana raisins**

½ cup (125 ml) **walnut or pecan crumbled**

1 tsp ground cinnamon

2 tsp vanilla extract

Pastry: Sift flour onto a clean flat surface and sprinkle with salt. Make a 1" (2.5 cm) dent in the flour and add egg yolk and 2 tablespoons of butter. Mix with your hands until crumbly. Add milk and mix again until dense and smooth. Place dough in plastic wrap and refrigerate 1 to 3 hours. Let dough sit for 20 minutes at room temperature then add 2 tablespoons of butter and knead.

Grease a 12" (30 cm) pie plate with butter and dust with flour. Cut a piece of parchment paper 14" (35 cm) wide. Preheat oven to 375°F (190°C).

Dust a clean flat surface with flour and roll out the dough until ½" (1 cm) thick and 14" (35 cm) across. Place dough in the pie plate, fluting the edges or pressing with a fork. Prick the dough on the bottom and sides with a fork so the pastry doesn't bubble when baking. Place parchment paper over the dough and fill with uncooked chickpeas. Blind bake the crust in the oven for 10 minutes then remove from oven and carefully remove parchment paper and chickpeas.

Filling: Peel, core and cut 6 apples in chunks. In a pan, sauté apple chunks with maple syrup, butter, raisins, walnut, cinnamon and vanilla until soft.

To assemble: Peel, core and thinly slice 2 apples. Using a slotted spoon, scoop filling into pastry then arrange apple slices on the top edge in a fan. Drizzle liquid from the pan over apple slices then bake in the oven for another 10 minutes.

Serves 8 to 10

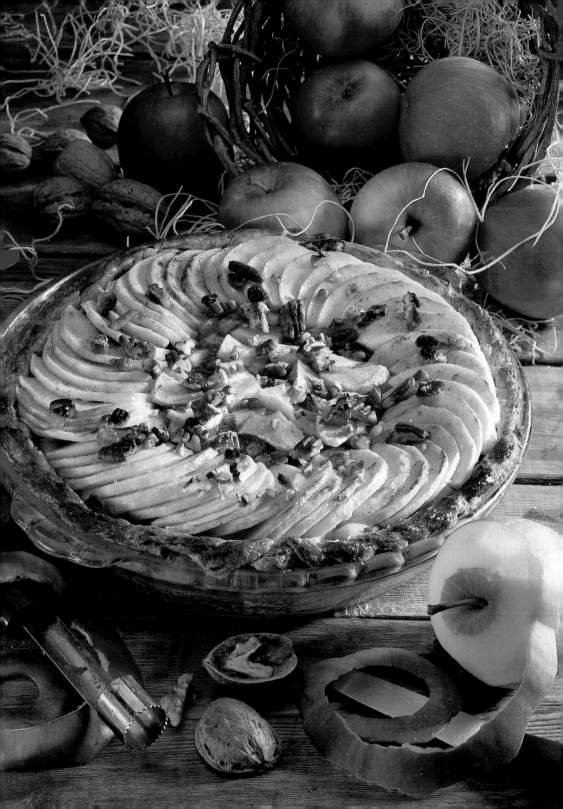

Coconut Banana

Banana is an energy booster that's been around for thousands of years. It was discovered in tropical countries and as humans found out how valuable this fruit was for nutrition, health and diet, we also discovered different kinds of medicinal uses for the whole plant—even the skin and leaves are used in natural medicine. Amazon doctors use banana leaf to cover the wound of the warriors and speed healing.

2 bananas, cut lengthwise in half and in 3" strips

1 tbsp butter

1 ½ tbsp maple syrup, Sucanat or Rapadura

¼ cup (60 ml) **coconut, shredded**

1 tsp sesame seeds

Melt butter in a saucepan (don't let it burn) then add banana and maple syrup and sauté for 3 to 4 minutes or until golden brown but not too soft. Add coconut and sesame seed; serve warm with vanilla ice cream, whipping cream or vanilla sauce.
Serves 2

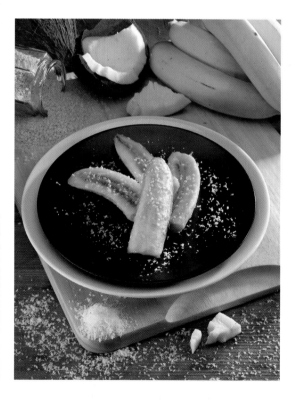

You can use baby bananas, they are more starchy and sweeter with more flavor and aroma. Banana comes in many different forms—popular types are baby banana, wild banana from India, and the regular banana. The plantain is one of the most used foods in the South American diet. Plantain flesh is firm and not as tasty as regular bananas.

references

Applied Nutrition Course, lessons 5 & 9, *alive* Academy of Nutrition, Burnaby, BC: *alive* books, 1993.

Ballentine, Rudolph. *Transition to Vegetarianism.* Honesdale, PA: Himalayan International Institute, 1987.

Bruder, Roy. *Discovering Natural Foods.* Santa Barbara, CA: Woodbridge Press, 1982.

Erasmus, Udo. *Fats That Heal, Fats That Kill.* Burnaby, BC: *alive* books, 1993

Heimlich, Jane. *What Your Doctor Won't Tell You.* New York: Harper Perennial, 1990.

Olinekova, Gayle. *Power Aging.* New York: Thunder's Mouth Press, 1998.

sources

for healthy oils:

Flora
7400 Fraser Park Drive
Burnaby BC V5J 5B9
(604) 436–6000
1-800–663–0617
(Western Canada)
1-800–387–7541
(Eastern Canada)

Omega-Life Inc.
15355 Woodridge Rd.
Brookfield, WI 53005
414-786-2070

Omega Nutrition of Canada Inc.
1924 Franklin Street
Vancouver, BC V5L 1R2
(604) 253-4677
1-800-661-3529
www.omegaflo.com

Barlean's
4936 Lake Terrell Road
Ferndale, WA 98248
(360)-384-0485
Orders: 1-800-445-3529
Fax: 1-800-551-9879

for kefir maker:

Teldon of Canada Ltd.
7434 Fraser Park Drive
Burnaby, BC V5J 5B9
Phone: (604) 436-0545
Orders: 1-800-663-2212
Fax: (604) 435-4862
E-mail: teldon@ultranet.ca

Remedies and supplements mentioned in this book are available at quality health food stores and nutrition centers.

First published in 2001 by
alive books
7436 Fraser Park Drive
Burnaby BC V5J 5B9
(604) 435–1919
1-800–661–0303

© 2001 by *alive* books

Book Design:
Liza Novecoski
Artwork:
Terence Yeung
Raymond Cheung
Food Styling/Recipe Development:
Fred Edrissi
Recipe Photos:
Edmond Fong
Cover Photo:
Edmond Fong
Photo Editing:
Sabine Edrissi-Bredenbrock
Editing:
Sandra Tonn

Canadian Cataloguing in Publication Data

Kathleen O'Bannon, CNC
Whole Foods for Seniors

(*alive* Natural Health Guides, 31
ISSN 1490-6503)
ISBN 1-55312-030-2

Printed in Canada

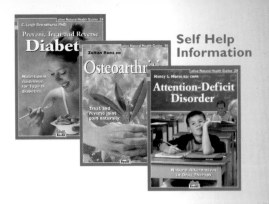
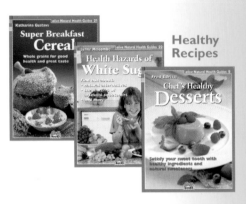
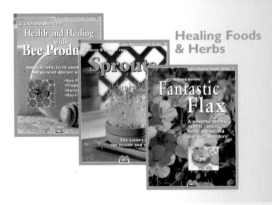
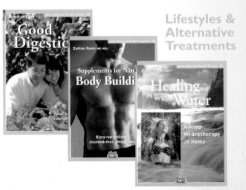